CDF

The Wellness Playbook

Consistency, Discipline, Focus

JAMES "CHIVO" GOLTL JR.

PIVOTT

PIAOTT Publishing
piaottpublishing@gmail.com
Chicago, Illinois

Print ISBN: 979-8-218-74254-6

To my son JC,

You are the heartbeat of my journey, the reason I push through the early mornings, the long workouts, and the toughest days. At just 10 years old, you've already shown more strength, support, and encouragement than most ever will.

You believe in me, your constant cheering, and the way you look up at me, even when I stumble, have been the fuel I didn't know I needed. Thank you for reminding me why this matters. Thank you for your high fives, the "'You got this, dad," moments, and your silent presence that tells me never to give up.

This journey is mine, but the reason behind it is you. You are smart, you are capable, and you are the best! With all my love and pride.

Dadda

Table of Contents

Intro...

Hitting your mid-30s, 40s, and 50s used to feel like the beginning of the end. Like you were sliding into dad-bod territory and midlife autopilot, but nah, that old script's dead. These days, your midlife can be your second prime. You've got muscle, mindset, and now mileage. It's all coming together.

Now, real talk: For a lot of dudes, this decade hits different. Your metabolism? Slows down. Hangovers? Last two days. Energy? Not what it used to be. Those health red flags you've been ignoring? Yeah, they start knocking. But this isn't the time to throw in the towel; it's the time to boss up, get off your ass, handle your business, and get to work.

Being healthy in your midlife isn't about chasing your 20s. It's about being strong, sharp, and unshakable. Being healthy is for you, your people, your grind, and the life you're still out here trying to live to the fullest.

Whether you're just now getting serious about your health or you've been at it and want to hit that next level, this book's got you covered.

We're talking fitness, food, sleep, stress, and mindset. The whole package. Remember! This point in your life isn't about looking young, but if looking young happens, that's a bonus. It's about feeling powerful, strong, and confident. Let's make this time in your life the launchpad, and not the slow fade.

It's never too late to build strength, work on your mental well-being, and get your health back on track. It's time to lock in and get to work!

Common Health Challenges for Men

1. Weight Gain & Slower Metabolism?

Let's keep it 100. Once you hit a certain age, that belly starts showing up like it's got an invite. Even if you're eating the same and hitting the gym here and there, the scale still creeps up. Your Testosterone levels drop, metabolism slows down, and suddenly that second slice of pizza sticks around a little longer, and those love handles start to get a little bigger. Those shirts start getting a little snug, and your pants are getting tighter.

2. Losing Muscle Like Loose Change?

Muscle starts dipping on you, quietly. It's called sarcopenia, and it kicks off in your 40s. If you're not lifting or doing something to fight back, fat starts moving in where muscle used to live. Strength drops, posture slouches, and your whole system starts slowing down.

3. "Low T" Isn't Just a Buzzword?

Testosterone doesn't just fall off a cliff, but it does take a slow dive. About 1% a year after 30. By your 40s, you might start feeling it: Low sex drive, low energy, mood swings, harder to build muscle, and you really don't feel like yourself. Not every guy gets hit hard, but a lot of us start noticing something's off.

4. Stress Is No Joke?

Let's be real, life comes with a full plate the older you get: career grind, bills, relationships, kids, aging parents. Everything starts to pile up. And too many of us are still stuck in that "just suck it up" mindset because that's what we've been told our whole life as men. But ignoring it does you no good. That's how you slide into anxiety, burnout, and sleepless nights. Mental health matters.

5. Sleep Be Acting Funny?

Sleep isn't what it used to be. Hormones change, stress builds, and next thing you know, you're staring at the ceiling at 3 AM. Too much caffeine, late-night scrolling, or drinks before bed just make it worse. Sleep apnea, snoring, or plain old insomnia, or hell, you have to get up in the middle of the night and go piss, whatever it is, it drags everything else down with it.

6. Skipping The Doctor Like It's Optional?

A bunch of guys haven't seen a doctor in years. No judgment! We all think we're fine until something breaks. Now's the time to lock in those checkups, get your blood work done, and handle the screenings. Don't wait until your body starts yelling at you and breaking down.

How It Started
My Wake-Up Call

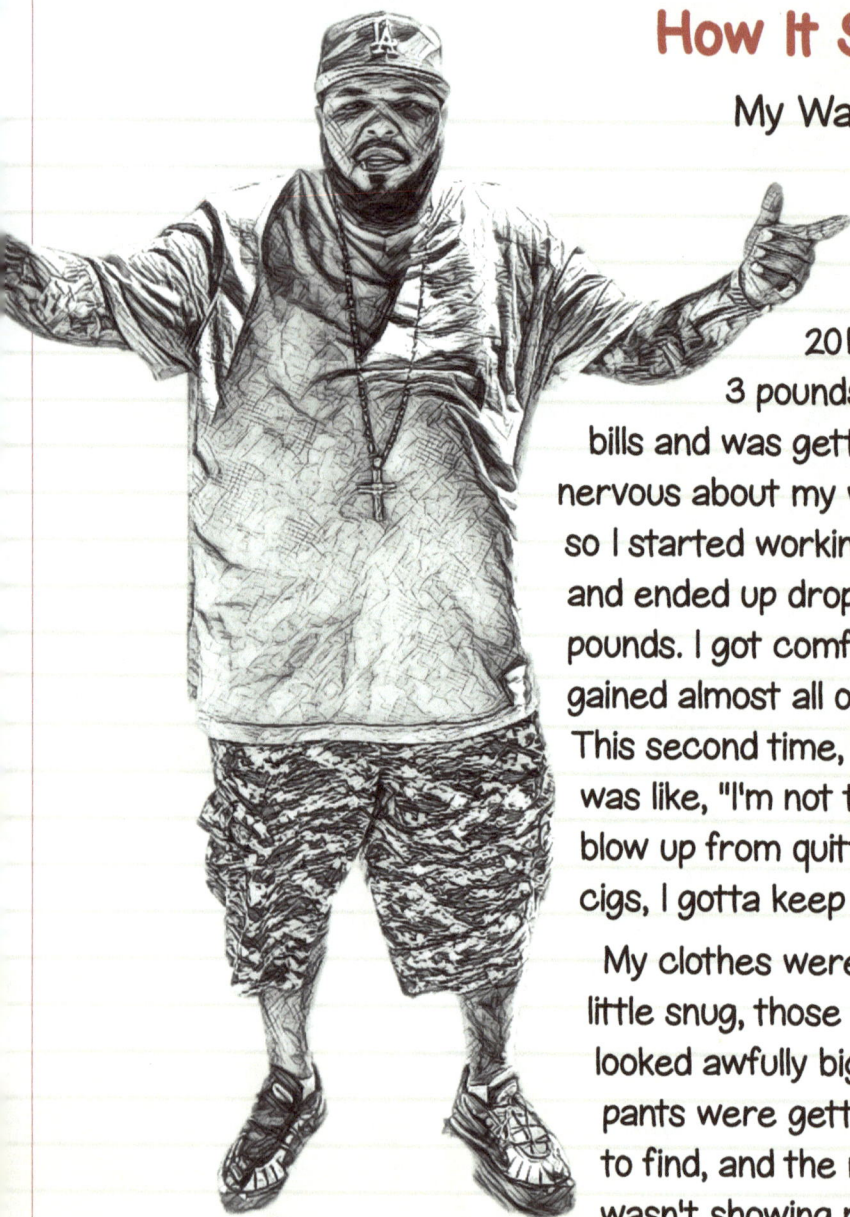

Back in 2012, I was 3 pounds shy of 3 bills and was getting a little nervous about my weight, so I started working out and ended up dropping 103 pounds. I got comfortable and gained almost all of it back. This second time, though, I was like, "I'm not trying to blow up from quitting these cigs, I gotta keep it tight."

My clothes were feeling a little snug, those 4x shirts looked awfully big, the 44 pants were getting hard to find, and the mirror wasn't showing me any love. Straight throwing shade every time I looked into it.

When I first started, I was just looking to lose around 50, to go from 289 to around 230/235, but once I got in the zone, it was a wrap. The pounds started flying off like nothing. I lost 74 pounds in three months.

Five years back, right after Mother's Day, I made the hardest and best decision of my life: I quit drinking. I was what they call a "functional alcoholic," but inside? I was crashing. I was an angry drunk, very argumentative, just plain ol' mean! Only a few people knew how bad my drinking was. I was locked in. It had become part of my daily routine, but I knew I had to stop; not just for me, but for my son. I got into a bad argument with someone I was close to, and the next day I told myself I was done drinking.

I stopped smoking on April 9th, two weeks after that, I started working out, and the day after Mother's Day, I stopped drinking. So, within a little over a month, I decided to do all these things at one time.

It was the smoking that was hard. But I would put myself in situations where I would be around cigarette smoke to challenge myself to see if I would stay solid or slip.

I did the same when I was drinking. Hit the bars with the homies, grabbed water while they sipped brews, and when they had shots, I had my own shot glass, just filled it up with sugar-free energy drink, so I was taking shots right along with 'em. Except mine was giving me a different kind of boost. I always liked to challenge myself, even before all this health stuff. I would stop drinking for two months just to see who was in control, me or the alcohol.

I took that same energy I was using to drink and flipped it into taking care of myself, started eating cleaner, and moving smarter. Still got the receipts too; the scale said 289 back then. Let me tell you how my headspace flipped. I could be having the worst day, but once I hit a run, hop on the bike, or just step out in the fresh air, man, it's like instant peace.

Watching planes fly low over my head, birds chirping, wind hitting my face, man, that sun hits different when your mind's heavy. Nothing like it. Best thing for your mental health. If you want to shake off some stress, start tossing around some weights. Weights are way better than going home, cracking a bottle, and sitting in that dark cloud.

The early days were rough, no lie. But I found my way out through the gym. The workouts gave me purpose; Gave me peace. I traded the bottle for the barbell, and I've never looked back.

Bottom line, your mid-30s, 40s, and 50s, isn't the end; it's the reset. You can either coast or take control. Let's build, not break

The Mental Mindset

It Isn't Just Your Body That Has To Level Up! It's Your Mindset Too.

This isn't the decade for "grind till you drop." That hustle-hard mentality? It starts to backfire. Now it's all about working smarter, not harder. Health isn't about ego anymore; it's about being consistent, disciplined, and focused.

1. Ditch Motivation. Lock in Discipline

Back in your 20s or 30s, you could ride that hype wave. Get fired up, hit the gym, skip meals, bounce back quickly. But now? Life's stacked; kids, work, bills, stress. If you're waiting on motivation, you'll be waiting forever.

New mindset: I don't need to feel like it, I just do it.

Make it automatic. Meal prep. Set your workout schedule like a meeting. Block off sleep. Discipline holds you down when the hype fades.

2. Redefine Winning

Six-pack? Cool. Heavy bench? Respect.

But focus on real wins now. Waking up without pain. Having energy for your kids. Staying sharp in meetings. Feeling good in your own skin.

New mindset: Fitness is fuel. Not my whole identity.

Train to live better, not just to flex. Make moves that actually serve your lifestyle, not your ego.

3. Train Smarter, Not Just Harder

You're not broken, but you're not made of rubber anymore either. Injuries hit harder. Recovery takes longer. You can still go hard, but do it with purpose.

New mindset: I'm training to still be a beast at 60.

Mobility. Rest. Smart programming. It's not soft, it's strategy. Play the long game.

4. Kill the All-or-Nothing Trap

Missed a workout? Had a rough weekend? Ate like trash? It happens. Doesn't mean it's over. Stop thinking you have to be perfect. Just don't quit. Stay consistent.

New Mindset: One move forward is better than none.

20-minute walk? That counts. One healthy meal? Still a win. Keep showing up. It adds up. Try to maintain consistency.

5. Lead With Your Health

People are watching even when you don't notice; Your kids. Your homies. Your coworkers. Being healthy isn't selfish; it's leadership.

New mindset: How I show up for myself is how I show up for others.

Set the tone. Be the example. Take care of yourself, so you can take care of what matters.

6. Stay Hungry, Stay Sharp

The biggest danger now isn't failure, it's settling, going on autopilot, and getting soft. Don't let midlife be your slow fade. Let it be the new you.

New mindset: I'm not done. I'm just getting started.

Read. Try new things. Evolve. Surround yourself with real ones who push you forward.

Bottom Line? This isn't a midlife crisis, it's a midlife come-up. Play smart. Stay sharp. Keep building.

YOU'VE GOT WAY MORE IN THE TANK.

Date: _____ Current Mindset: _____

_____

_____

_____

_____

_____

_____

_____

Some Daily Hype Talk for You

Lock In!

Say it in the mirror. Whisper it mid-set while you're working out. Scream it if that works. Write it on a sticky note. These aren't just words; this is how you rewire your mindset, change your vibe, and flip your subconscious mind.

Mindset + Identity

"I'm not washed up! I'm just warming up."

"I move with a mission, not for clout."

"Every rep's makin' me a beast version of me."

"This is my king era."

"I'm not trying to be who I was. I'm building someone better."

Discipline + Consistency

"Even when I don't want to, I show up."

"I don't make excuses. I make progress."

"Stacking small wins turns into big flexes."

"Mind strong. Body stronger. I'm built for this."

"Perfection's fake. I just keep it moving."

Confidence + Energy

"I walk like I lift. I speak like I mean it."

"My grind shows. I don't have to brag."

"How I train is how I live. All gas." No breaks!

"I'm not just talking, I'm doing."

"I got the juice. And I prove it daily."

Focus + Self-Respect

"L's don't stop me! They teach me."

"Every scar's a stripe. Every rep's earned."

"Motivation fades, standards don't."

"I'm not here to impress. I'm here to evolve."

"If I don't respect me, who will?"

REAL ONES KNOW:

Say it out loud. Chest up, voice firm. Slap three on your mirror, let 'em hit every morning.

Pick a different one every workout and let it ride in your head until you're finished.

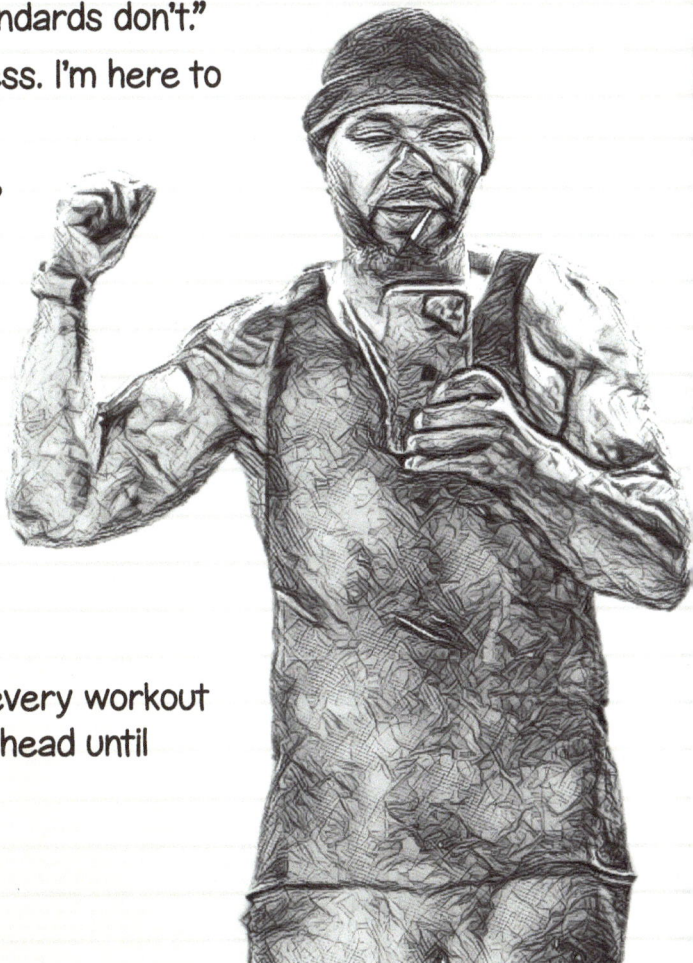

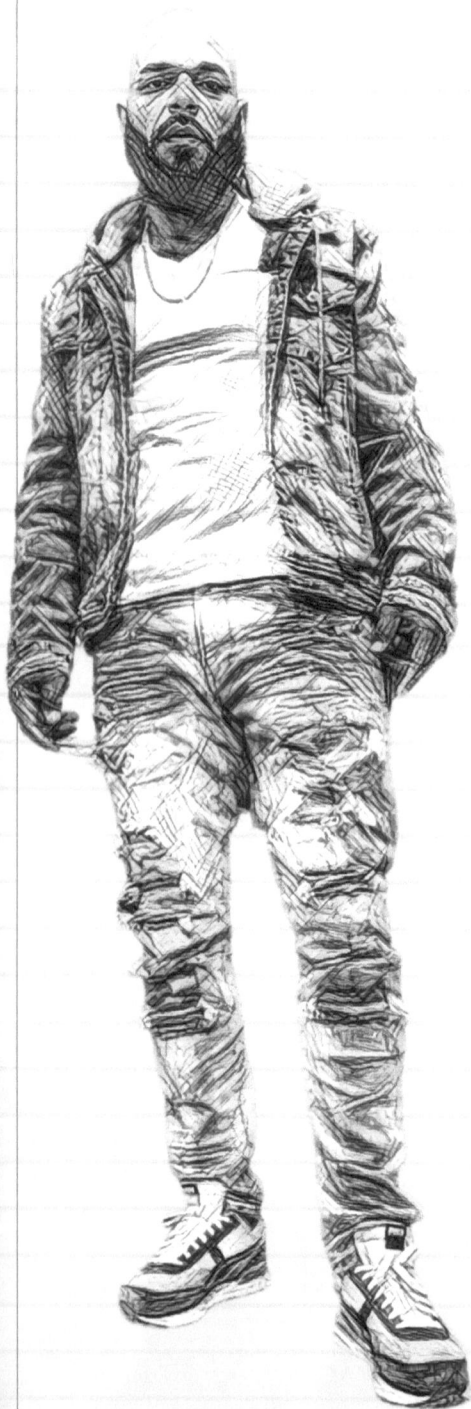

"Train to be strong.
Move to stay young.
Rest to bounce back."

–Chivo

Building a Balanced Fitness Routine

This Isn't The Endgame. This Is The Come-Up.

Your body's still got gas in the tank; Strength, speed, endurance, it's all there. Here's the truth, though. Recovery's slower, injuries hit harder, and you can't be out here training like you're 25 anymore.

Now it's all about balance. Push hard, but train smart. Build muscle, stay mobile, keep the heart pumping, and play the long game.

The Game Plan

Train smart, not reckless. Recovery is just as important as your grind. Mix it up: strength, cardio, mobility, flexibility.

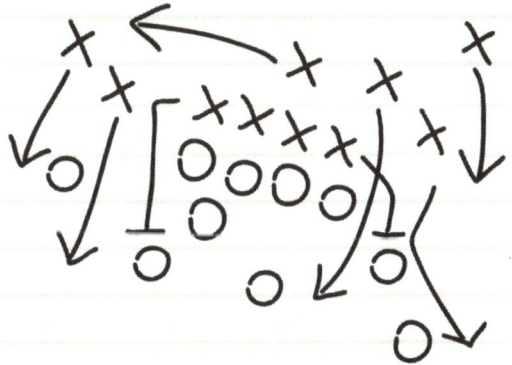

I. STRENGTH TRAINING (4X A WEEK)	
Muscle isn't just for looks, they keep your metabolism humming, your joints solid, and your hormones happy.	
Choose your split:	Option A: Full body lifts every other day
	Option B: Push/Pull/Legs or Upper/Lower split

1. STRENGTH TRAINING (4X A WEEK)

Focus on the good stuff!	Big lifts:	Squats, deadlifts, presses, pull-ups, rows
	Core moves:	Planks, bird-dogs, dead bugs, bicycle crunches Medium weight, slow and controlled reps.
Reps:		6-12 per set
Sets:		2-4

Pro tip: Warm up right, dial in your form, and every 6-8 weeks, take a de-load week to let the body reset.

2. CARDIO & HEART HEALTH

You need to keep that engine running clean. Cardio isn't just about fat burn, it's about longevity.

1x a week	Strictly cardio
4X a week - 30 min.	Treadmill, an incline or outdoor walk (After workout)
Your options:	Zone 2 work: brisk walk, light jog, or bike ride. 30-45 min., chill pace. Fun stuff: sports, hiking, swimming, whatever keeps you moving.
Hit these (1 to 2x week):	Sprints, circuits, dumbbell, kettle bells short and hard, 30 to 40 minutes.

Quick and efficient time conserving workouts to do when you're short on time and want to switch up from a traditional workout. Burn a lot of calories in a short amount of time.

Pro tip: Don't train to the point of collapse. Stay consistent and recover hard.

3. MOBILITY & FLEXIBILITY (EVERY DAY OR AS NEEDED)

Mobility is your secret weapon. Keeps the joints smooth, prevents tweaks, helps you bounce back quicker.

Hit these regularly:	Hip openers, T-spine rotations, shoulder drills
	Stretch flows or yoga (10-20 min. daily or post-lift)
	Foam roll or grab a lacrosse ball and hit those tight spots

Pro tip: Just 5-10 min. a day adds up. Don't sleep on it.

4. RECOVERY & REST

Don't be that guy who trains hard but skips sleep. Rest is where the real gains happen.

Daily:	Aim for 7-8 hours of solid sleep.
Once per week:	Take at least one full rest day
Try active recovery:	Light walks, sauna, gentle stretching

Day	Focus
Mon	Strength (Push Upper Body)
Tues	Zone 2 Cardio + Mobility + Core
Wed	Strength (Pull Upper Body)
Thurs	HIT or Sports + Flexibility
Fri	Strength (Lower Body)
Sat	HIT workout (full body kettle bell or dumbbell)
Sun	Rest or Gentle Yoga

Hey! This time in your life isn't about dialing it down. It's about training smarter than ever. You don't have to kill yourself in the gym. Just stay consistent, intentional, and well-rounded. Train to be strong, move to stay young, and rest to bounce back.

Play the long game, and your 30s, 40s, and 50s might just be your strongest years yet. Trust the process and not the timeline. Don't trip if the scale isn't moving fast. Don't stress if your homie is further ahead. This is your lane. Your race. Your damn story. Respect the slow wins because that's where the growth lives.

Keep Stepping. This journey isn't about perfection; it's about showing up when it's hard, staying solid when you plateau, and never letting comfort kill progress. So lace up, lift up, and level up. You're not falling off, you're rising back up. Day by day. Brick by brick.

LET'S GET IT!

Weight Management and Why It Matters More Than Ever

Weight Gain in Mid-life is Built Different

Yo, managing your weight isn't about starving yourself or grinding 24/7; it's about moving smart, eating with purpose, and stacking habits that stick. Let's break it down:

Lifting Is Mandatory, Not Optional

Muscle is your secret weapon. It keeps your metabolism lit and your body running lean, even when you're chilling.

Hit the weights 3x a week. NO EXCUSES.

Stick to the heavy hitters: squats, deadlifts, presses, and pull-ups.

Full-body workouts over chasing pump days.

Muscles burn more calories, even at rest.

Protein Is the Plug

Do you want to keep muscle, stay full, and avoid late-night snack attacks? Protein's your best friend.

Shoot for 0.7g of protein per pound of your goal weight.

Include it in every meal: eggs, chicken, salmon, lentils, Greek yogurt, protein shakes, or whatever suits your taste.

More protein = less munching = leaner you.

Casein protein before bed is your friend.

Eat Smart, Not Perfect

Forget crash diets and weird trends. Weight management

is about playing the long game.

Cut down on the junk: less sugar, less processed trash. Stack your plate with protein, good fats, and fiber-rich carbs.

Follow the 80/20 rule: eat clean 80% of the time and enjoy life the other 20%.

<u>Pro tip:</u> Track your food for a week; you're probably eating more than you think, especially on weekends with the sneaky bites.

Get a calorie tracker app. Count Macros, not Calories.

Keep Booze & Liquid Calories in Check

Alcohol hits different. It wrecks your sleep, messes with Testosterone levels, and packs on sneaky pounds.

Keep it light: 1-2 drinks a week if you must, or go dry and feel the glow.

Ditch the sugar bombs: no soda, no energy drinks, no fancy "healthy" juices.

Stick to water, black coffee, and unsweetened tea. Hydrate like a boss.

Sleep Like It's Your Job, Stress Like You Give a Damn

You can lift, eat clean, and still fall off if your sleep is trash and your stress is wild.

Lock in 7-8 hours a night. non-negotiable

Chill your mind: deep breaths, walks, journaling, therapy,

hobbies, or whatever keeps you cool.

Less stress = less fat storage = better vibes all around

Consistency Over Perfection

Forget going 100% for a week. Go 70-80% forever. The wins come from consistency, not hacks.

Think years, not weeks.

Build a lifestyle you can ride with at 50, 60, 70+

You're not trying to "look good for summer," you're trying to feel good for life.

Mindset Shift: The Health Scale

Don't chase a number. Chase how you feel, move, and show up.

Remember! Smaller waistline. Smaller scale number.

Trade fat for muscle and feel like a beast.

Better sleep, energy, mood, and strength. That's the real blow-up.

Embrace the Grind

This fitness journey is not just about gains; it's a grind. A lifestyle. A full-blown comeback.

The real ones are not scared of the slow climb. We respect it.

Look, fam! Getting fit isn't a sprint. It's not about quick fixes, magic shakes, or overnight six-pack dreams. Getting fit is not just about willpower; it's about the blueprint.

Design your days, and build habits that stick. Play the long game because with the right mix of training, fuel, sleep, and mindset, you'll stay lean, strong, and locked-in for decades.

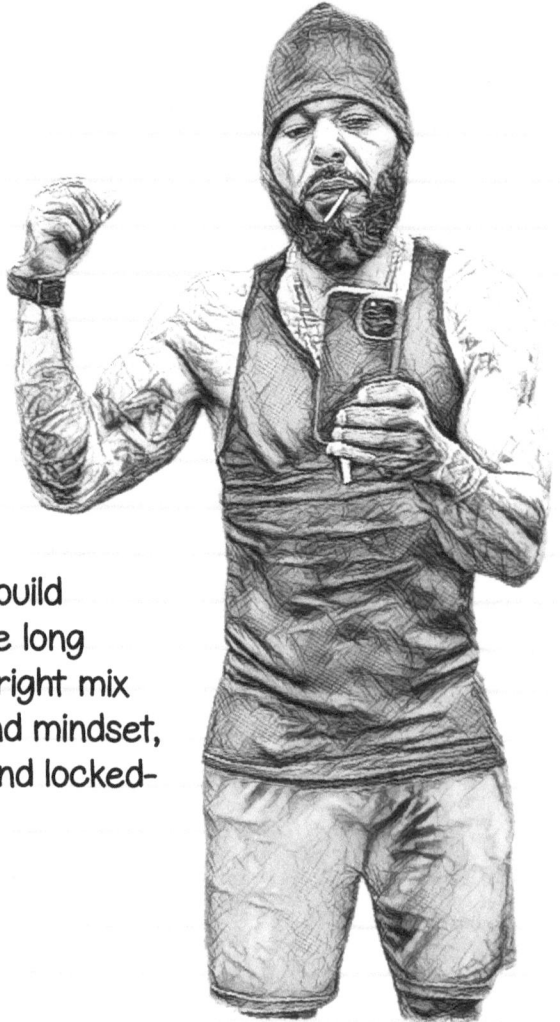

What's the first bad habit you need to break?

_____

_____

_____

_____

_____

_____

_____

Eating Healthy Fuel for Strength, Energy, and Longevity
Eat Like You Mean It!

So listen, your body isn't letting you slide with late-night pizza and gas station snacks like it used to. You're not just eating to flex in the gym anymore; you're eating to protect your health, keep your muscle, keep your hormones in check, and stay mentally sharp. What you're about to learn isn't diet culture. It's a strategy.

Why Life Hits Different Now:

Slow-ass metabolism: You burn less just chilling, so what you eat matters way more.

Muscle matters: Gotta fight to keep that lean mass up.

Hormone shift: Testosterone levels, insulin, cortisol; all of them are tied to what's on your plate.

Inflammation creeping in: Junk food hits your joints, energy, and focus. Clean eating helps you bounce back.

1. Protein Has To Be Front and Center

No more sidepiece protein. Make it the main character.

Goal: 0.7g per pound of your GOAL weight.

Get it from: Eggs, chicken, Greek yogurt, shakes, fish, tofu, lentils.

Example: If you want to weigh 180, aim for or at least 180g of protein a day.

Pro tip: Every plate needs protein.

2. Eat Real Food, Not Fake Crap.

If it's in a shiny wrapper and lasts 6 months, it's bad.

STACK UP

Veggies for fiber and nutrients

Fruits (especially berries and citrus)

Whole grains like oats, rice, and quinoa

Healthy fats from nuts, seeds, olive oil, and fatty fish

Pro tip: Eat the rainbow. More color = more benefits.

3. Carbs Aren't All Evil, Just Be Smart With Them.

You don't need to dismiss carbs, just manage the relationship better.

Rock with: Sweet potatoes, fruit, lentils, brown rice

Skip: White bread, candy, donuts, sugary cereal

The best time to eat carbs is around workouts or when you're moving.

Pro tip: If you're not active that day, lean on veggies, protein, and healthy fats for fuel.

4. Fat Is Your Friend. Just Don't Wild Out.

Good fats = healthy hormones and a happy brain.

Eat: Avocados, olive oil, salmon, nuts, seeds.

Just don't overdo it. These fats are dense, so keep the servings light.

Pro tip: Fat doesn't make you fat, eating like it's Thanksgiving every day does.

5. Water Still Runs the Show.

Dehydration is a sneaky villain. It kills your vibe, focus, and even your cravings.

Goal: 3-4 liters a day (100-130 oz.)

Drink more water if you're sweating, working out, or drinking caffeine/alcohol.

Pro tip: Start your day with 2 glasses of water before that coffee hits your lips.

6. Cut the Crap That Drags You Down.

Do you want to feel better, sleep better, and keep your hormones steady? Ease up on the trash.

Booze kills your testosterone, wrecks your sleep, and adds empty calories.

Sugar = cravings, crashes, and chubby gains.

Processed foods = trash macros, no value.

Late-night stuffing = messed-up sleep and digestion.

Pro tip: If you wouldn't feed it to your kid, don't feed it to your damn self.

7. What a Day Could Look Like

Here's how clean eating can still slap:

Breakfast: 3 eggs, avocado, sautéed spinach, berries

Lunch: Grilled chicken salad, olive oil dressing, side of sweet potatoes.

Snack: Greek yogurt + almonds or a protein shake.

Dinner: Salmon, roasted veggies, quinoa.

Optional: Square of dark chocolate or herbal tea before bed or Greek yogurt with berries.

Eating like this isn't about being perfect; it's about eating with purpose. You're not chasing six-packs, you're building a body that holds up strong and sharp for the next 40 years Healthy food is fuel to feel good. Fuel to stay sharp. Fuel to stay strong.

YOU'RE GROWN NOW. EAT LIKE IT.

How do you feel at this point about healthy eating?

_____

_____

_____

_____

_____

_____

_____

_____

_____

_____

Smart Lifestyle Choice
Midlife = Fork in the Road

This decade is a crossroads. You either slide into that slow decline, or step up, lock in, and build the blueprint for your best years. Real talk! A few consistent tweaks right now can slash your risk of disease, crank up your energy, and keep you feeling solid, strong, and sharp every day.

1. Sleep isn't Optional. It's Your Superpower.

Want to feel good, perform better, and stay lean? Get your sleep game right.

Goal: 7-8 hours of solid sleep.

Dial it in: Stick to the same sleep/wake times, use a blackout room, maintain a cool temperature, and avoid screens before bed.

Why it matters: Trash sleep = weight gain, low T, heart problems, and brain fog.

Real tip: Treat bedtime like a boss meeting. It's that important.

2. Move More! Gym or Not.

Yeah, the workouts matter, but it's the everyday movement that stacks up.

Goal: 8k-10k steps daily, plus 3-5 workouts per week.

Add: Walk breaks, stairs, stretches in the morning.

Why: That NEAT movement (non-exercise stuff) boosts

your burn, joints, and vibe.

Real tip: You can't out-train a couch. Get up and move more, period.

3. Ease Up on the Booze

Alcohol hits different. Booze hurts your sleep, weakens your recovery, and causes hormone dips.

Try: Keep it to 1-2 drinks a week, or go dry and see what's up.

Red flag: "One drink" turning into a nightly routine messes with your focus.

Real tip: Go 30 days off. I bet you'll sleep better, think clearer, and feel lighter.

4. Handle Your Stress Like a Grown Man

Stress isn't just annoying, it's wrecking your body if you don't manage it.

Tools that work: Walks

Breathwork / meditation (5-10 min)

Lifting weights (built-in stress relief)

Laughing, hobbies, kickin' it with good people.

Real tip: Managing stress isn't a luxury; it's part of the health grind now.

5. Check Under the Hood

Don't wait for stuff on your body to break before you act.

Prevention = power.

Stay on top of: Blood pressure, cholesterol, blood sugar

Hormone levels, especially Testosterone.

Colon checks. (Starts at 45.)

Prostate health.

Mental health too, no shame in that.

Real tip: Know your numbers. Early checks save lives.

6. Invest in Your People

Are you "too busy" for real connections? That's how dudes end up burnt out and alone.

Put energy into: Your relationship.

Close friends.

Mentors and people who uplift.

Be real, be open. Connection is
not a weakness, it's protection.

Real tip: Strong men build tribes; they don't go lone wolf.

7. Train Your Brain Too

Being fit is not just about your biceps. Your brain needs reps, too.

Read books.

Try new skills or hobbies.

Cut the doom-scrolling.

Journal or write your thoughts out.

Real tip: Keep your mind sharp. Can't flex if you're foggy upstairs.

8. Set Up Your Space to Win

Your environment = your autopilot. Make it work for you, not against you.

Stock the fridge with good eats.

Create screen-time & work boundaries.

Hang with folks who actually care about growth.

Real tip: Build a space that backs up your goals, not tempts your excuses.

Again, midlife doesn't have to be a slow fade. Midlife can be the take-off point, especially if you show up with intention. Sleep better, eat smarter, move more, stress less, and lock in with good people. Again, it's not about perfection; it's about showing up on purpose.

Health is a lifestyle now. Own it.

Conclusion

By now, you've seen some things. You know what matters, what's noise, and the kind of man you're trying to be. Your health? It's gotta match that wisdom.

Being strong isn't just about muscle.

Health isn't just numbers on a chart.

It's about showing up with energy, focus, and purpose. For your family, your hustle, your life.

IT'S ABOUT OWNERSHIP

This chapter's all about owning your life:

Own your habits

Own your mindset

Own your future

You don't have to be perfect. Just show up on the regular.

You're not chasing the past. You're building a future that hits different in every decade. **The Real Win?**

It isn't just about looking good in the mirror, it's about:

Feeling dialed in.

Moving with power.

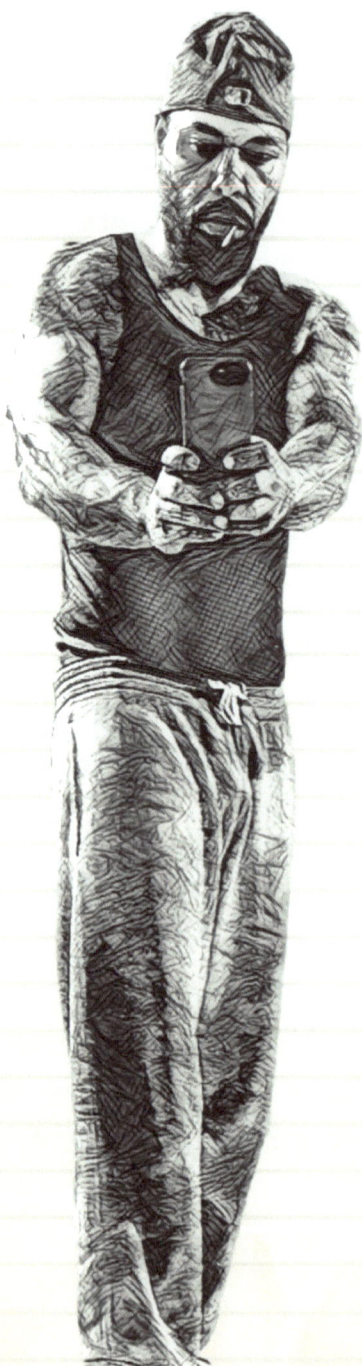

Living with clarity and confidence.

Every! Single! Day!

This Is Your Time.

This is the comeback season.

The lead-from-the-front era.

Time to:

Reclaim your body.

Upgrade your mind.

Lock in for the long haul.

YOUR BEST YEARS?

They're not behind you, they're just getting started.

LET'S GO.

The Check-In Journal

Alright, fellas, time for the "midlife check-in." But don't stress, this isn't your grandma's diary. I created a space for you to keep it real about your body, your mind, and everything in between. Write it all down. The good, the bad, and the ugly. This part is between you and you.

What's This?

The next few pages, journal's your spot to track the real stuff. The workouts, sleep, stress, mood, or whatever is going on. It's like a check-up without the doc. Stay sharp, feel better, keep moving. Here's my example:

My Check-In

Date:	June 2, 2025
Day of the Week:	Monday
I. PHYSICAL HEALTH	
Sleep:	
Hours slept:	7.5
Sleep quality:	(Out of 5)
Notes:	Woke up once during the night but fell back asleep easily.

Exercise:	
Activity:	30-minute brisk walk + bodyweight strength routine.
Energy level:	
Notes:	Felt strong during the workout. Stretching helped lower back tightness.
Diet & Nutrition:	
Meals:	Breakfast: Oatmeal with berries and almonds. Lunch: Grilled chicken salad. Dinner: Salmon, quinoa, and steamed veggies.
Water intake:	2.5L
Alcohol:	None
Notes:	Ate clean today. Craved sugar in the afternoon but had fruit instead.

2. MENTAL & EMOTIONAL WELLNESS

Mood:	Content
Stress Level:	3/10

Notes:	Work was manageable. It took 10 minutes for deep breathing mid-day, which helped focus.
Reflection/ Gratitude:	Today I'm grateful for: My sons' laughter at dinner. Reminded me not to take life too seriously.
Wins of the Day:	Finished a tough work presentation and stayed consistent with my workout.
Challenges:	I had a short fuse with a coworker this morning. Need to work on patience and not letting small things trigger frustration.

3. PREVENTIVE & LONG-TERM HEALTH

Medical Check-ins:

Blood pressure (if tracked):	122/78
Medications/ supplements:	Multivitamin, Omega-3
Any pain or symptoms:	Slight stiffness in right shoulder.

Health Goals for the Week:

Goal 1:	Get 7+ hours of sleep each night.

Goal 2:	Limit caffeine to 1 cup/day.
Goal 3:	Schedule annual physical.

4. PERSONAL GROWTH & LIFESTYLE

Reading/Podcasts:

Read/Listened to:	"The Drive" with Dr. Peter Attia - Episode on longevity
Insight:	Resistance training is one of the top predictors of longevity.

Relationships & Social Life:

Called an old friend. Planning a weekend hike with my brother.

Quote of the Day:

Take care of your body.
It's the only place you have to live.

We all have to start somewhere, and if you've never journaled before, here's a week's worth of pages to begin your new way of life. Keep up with your progress, write what you're feeling, and be open and honest. Remember, it's about you and your journey, so let the words flow freely. Use my reference only as a guide as you begin the process of regaining YOU again.

The Check-In

Day 1

Today's Motivation:	

Date:	
Day of the Week:	

I. PHYSICAL HEALTH

Sleep:

Hours slept:	
Sleep quality:	
Notes:	

Exercise:

Activity:	

Energy level:

Notes:	

Diet & Nutrition:	
Meals:	Breakfast: Lunch: Dinner:
Water intake:	
Alcohol:	
Notes:	

2. MENTAL & EMOTIONAL WELLNESS

Mood:	
Stress Level:	
Notes:	
Reflection/ Gratitude:	
Wins of the Day:	

Challenges:	

3. PREVENTIVE & LONG-TERM HEALTH

Medical Check-ins:

Blood pressure (if tracked):	
Medications/ supplements:	
Any pain or symptoms:	

Health Goals for the Week:

Goal 1:	
Goal 2:	
Goal 3:	

Extra info: _____
_____
_____
_____
_____
_____

4. PERSONAL GROWTH & LIFESTYLE

Reading/Podcasts:	
Read/Listened to:	
Insight:	

Relationships & Social Life:

Quote of the Day:

Notes:

_____

_____

_____

_____

_____

_____

_____

_____

_____

_____

The Check-In

Day 2

Today's Motivation:	

Date:	
Day of the Week:	

I. PHYSICAL HEALTH

Sleep:

Hours slept:	
Sleep quality:	
Notes:	

Exercise:

Activity:	

Energy level:

Notes:	

Diet & Nutrition:	
Meals:	Breakfast:
	Lunch:
	Dinner:
Water intake:	
Alcohol:	
Notes:	

2. MENTAL & EMOTIONAL WELLNESS

Mood:	
Stress Level:	
Notes:	
Reflection/ Gratitude:	
Wins of the Day:	

Challenges:	

3. PREVENTIVE & LONG-TERM HEALTH

Medical Check-ins:	
Blood pressure (if tracked):	
Medications/ supplements:	
Any pain or symptoms:	

Health Goals for the Week:	
Goal 1:	
Goal 2:	
Goal 3:	

Extra info: _____
_____
_____
_____
_____
_____

4. PERSONAL GROWTH & LIFESTYLE

Reading/Podcasts:

Read/Listened to:	
Insight:	

Relationships & Social Life:

Quote of the Day:

Notes: _____
_____
_____
_____
_____
_____
_____
_____
_____
_____

The Check-In

Day 3

Today's Motivation:	
Date:	
Day of the Week:	

<table>
<tr><td colspan="2" style="background-color:#b5524a; color:white; text-align:center">I. PHYSICAL HEALTH</td></tr>
<tr><td colspan="2" style="text-align:center">Sleep:</td></tr>
<tr><td>Hours slept:</td><td></td></tr>
<tr><td>Sleep quality:</td><td></td></tr>
<tr><td>Notes:</td><td></td></tr>
<tr><td colspan="2" style="text-align:center">Exercise:</td></tr>
<tr><td>Activity:</td><td></td></tr>
<tr><td colspan="2" style="text-align:center">Energy level:</td></tr>
<tr><td>Notes:</td><td></td></tr>
</table>

Diet & Nutrition:	
Meals:	Breakfast:
	Lunch:
	Dinner:
Water intake:	
Alcohol:	
Notes:	

2. MENTAL & EMOTIONAL WELLNESS

Mood:	
Stress Level:	
Notes:	
Reflection/ Gratitude:	
Wins of the Day:	

Challenges:	

3. PREVENTIVE & LONG-TERM HEALTH	

Medical Check-ins:	
Blood pressure (if tracked):	
Medications/ supplements:	
Any pain or symptoms:	

Health Goals for the Week:	
Goal 1:	
Goal 2:	
Goal 3:	

Extra info: _____

_____

_____

_____

_____

_____

4. PERSONAL GROWTH & LIFESTYLE

Reading/Podcasts:

Read/Listened to:	
Insight:	

Relationships & Social Life:

Quote of the Day:

Notes:

The Check-In

Day 4

Today's Motivation:	

Date:	
Day of the Week:	

I. PHYSICAL HEALTH

Sleep:	
Hours slept:	
Sleep quality:	
Notes:	

Exercise:	
Activity:	

Energy level:	
Notes:	

Diet & Nutrition:	
Meals:	Breakfast:
	Lunch:
	Dinner:
Water intake:	
Alcohol:	
Notes:	

2. MENTAL & EMOTIONAL WELLNESS

Mood:	
Stress Level:	
Notes:	
Reflection/ Gratitude:	
Wins of the Day:	

Challenges:	

3. PREVENTIVE & LONG-TERM HEALTH

Medical Check-ins:

Blood pressure (if tracked):	
Medications/ supplements:	
Any pain or symptoms:	

Health Goals for the Week:

Goal 1:	
Goal 2:	
Goal 3:	

Extra info: _____

_____

_____

_____

_____

_____

4. PERSONAL GROWTH & LIFESTYLE

Reading/Podcasts:

Read/Listened to:	
Insight:	

Relationships & Social Life:

Quote of the Day:

Notes: _____
_____
_____
_____
_____
_____
_____
_____
_____
_____

The Check-In

Day 5

Today's Motivation:	

Date:	
Day of the Week:	

I. PHYSICAL HEALTH

Sleep:

Hours slept:	
Sleep quality:	
Notes:	

Exercise:

Activity:	

Energy level:

Notes:	

Diet & Nutrition:	
Meals:	Breakfast: Lunch: Dinner:
Water intake:	
Alcohol:	
Notes:	

2. MENTAL & EMOTIONAL WELLNESS

Mood:	
Stress Level:	
Notes:	
Reflection/ Gratitude:	
Wins of the Day:	

Challenges:	

3. PREVENTIVE & LONG-TERM HEALTH

Medical Check-ins:

Blood pressure (if tracked):	
Medications/ supplements:	
Any pain or symptoms:	

Health Goals for the Week:

Goal 1:	
Goal 2:	
Goal 3:	

Extra info: _____

_____

_____

_____

_____

_____

4. PERSONAL GROWTH & LIFESTYLE

Reading/Podcasts:	
Read/Listened to:	
Insight:	

Relationships & Social Life:

Quote of the Day:

Notes: _____

_____

_____

_____

_____

_____

_____

_____

_____

_____

The Check-In
Day 6

Today's Motivation:	

Date:	
Day of the Week:	

Sleep:

Hours slept:	
Sleep quality:	
Notes:	

Exercise:

Activity:	

Energy level:

Notes:	

Diet & Nutrition:	
Meals:	Breakfast: Lunch: Dinner:
Water intake:	
Alcohol:	
Notes:	

2. MENTAL & EMOTIONAL WELLNESS

Mood:	
Stress Level:	
Notes:	
Reflection/ Gratitude:	
Wins of the Day:	

Challenges:	

Medical Check-ins:

Blood pressure (if tracked):	
Medications/ supplements:	
Any pain or symptoms:	

Health Goals for the Week:

Goal 1:	
Goal 2:	
Goal 3:	

Extra info: _____

_____

_____

_____

_____

4. PERSONAL GROWTH & LIFESTYLE

Reading/Podcasts:

Read/Listened to:	
Insight:	

Relationships & Social Life:

Quote of the Day:

Notes:

_____

_____

_____

_____

_____

_____

_____

_____

_____

The Check-In

Day 7

Today's Motivation:	

Date:	
Day of the Week:	

I. PHYSICAL HEALTH

Sleep:

Hours slept:	
Sleep quality:	
Notes:	

Exercise:

Activity:	

Energy level:

Notes:	

Diet & Nutrition:	
Meals:	Breakfast: Lunch: Dinner:
Water intake:	
Alcohol:	
Notes:	

2. MENTAL & EMOTIONAL WELLNESS

Mood:	
Stress Level:	
Notes:	
Reflection/ Gratitude:	
Wins of the Day:	

Challenges:	

3. PREVENTIVE & LONG-TERM HEALTH

Medical Check-ins:

Blood pressure (if tracked):	
Medications/ supplements:	
Any pain or symptoms:	

Health Goals for the Week:

Goal 1:	
Goal 2:	
Goal 3:	

Extra info: _____
_____
_____
_____
_____
_____

4. PERSONAL GROWTH & LIFESTYLE

Reading/Podcasts:

Read/Listened to:	
Insight:	

Relationships & Social Life:

Quote of the Day:

Notes:

_____
_____
_____
_____
_____
_____
_____
_____
_____
_____

NOTES:

NOTES:

NOTES:

About the Author

J. "Chivo" Goltl is a skilled steamfitter mechanic based in Omaha, Nebraska, and a passionate advocate for men's health, after years of navigating the physical demands of his trade. James took his health into his own hands; Researching, experimenting, and ultimately transforming his life through fitness, nutrition, and a holistic approach to wellness.

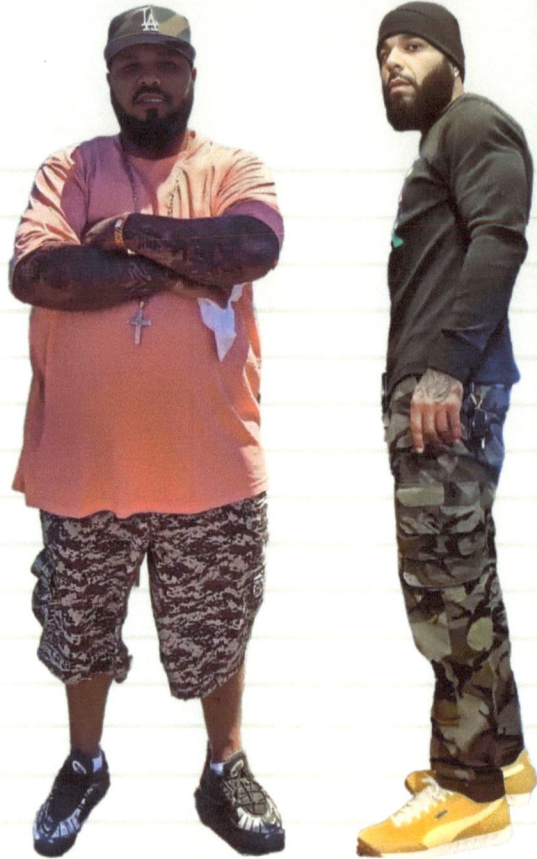

CDF The Wellness Playbook is his first book, written for men like him. Hardworking, driven, and ready to take back control of their bodies and lives. As a father to his son, JC, James is driven by a desire to create a lasting legacy and a sense of purpose. He recently won the OPPD Powering Holistic Health Leader Award, a testament to the impact of his journey and the wisdom he now shares.

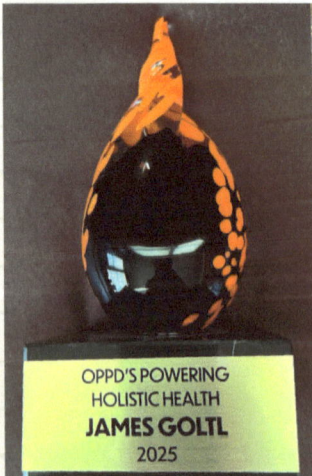

When he's not on the job or writing, you'll find him training at night, staying sharp in mind and body, and living proof that it's never too late to change your life.

OPPD'S POWERING
HOLISTIC HEALTH
JAMES GOLTL
2025

www.ingramcontent.com/pod-product-compliance
Lightning Source LLC
Chambersburg PA
CBHW041218270326
41931CB00001B/18